RED PILL SECRETS

Achieving status, Respect and Happiness through Traditional Masculinity

Kingsley Aneme

Email: Kingsleyaneme@gmail.com

Contact: +234 708 378 0104

Table of Content

INTRODUCTION

"Red Pill Philosophy

Chapter 1: Introduction to the "Red Pill" Philosophy

The phrase "red pill" is derived from the 1999 science fiction film The Matrix, in which the protagonist is given the option of taking a red pill, which would reveal the truth about the world, or a blue pill, which will enable him to continue living in ignorance. The phrase "red pill" is often used in current discourse to refer to a worldview that questions dominant views and encourages people to see the world as it really is, rather than how they have been conditioned to perceive it.

The "red pill" attitude is often linked to conventional masculinity and the notion that men should accept their natural responsibilities as leaders, providers, and guardians. Adherents of the "red pill" theory often contend that in contemporary times, traditional gender roles and cultural conventions have been twisted or abandoned, with detrimental implications for men and society as a whole.

The "red pill" ideology is fundamentally about individual responsibility and self-improvement. It empowers men to take charge of their life, create and accomplish objectives, and embrace their masculinity in a healthy and constructive manner.

Some of the key principles of the "red pill" philosophy include:

Personal responsibility: Men are responsible for their own actions and outcomes, and should take ownership of their lives rather than blaming external circumstances or other people.

- Hard work and self-improvement: Men should strive to continuously improve themselves, both physically and mentally, through hard work and dedication.

- Traditional gender roles: Men should embrace their natural roles as leaders, providers, and protectors, and women should embrace their natural roles as nurturers and caregivers.
- Rational thinking and objective truth: Men should strive to see the world as it really is, rather than being swayed by emotion or societal conditioning.
- Self-reliance: Men should be self-sufficient and capable of providing for themselves and their families.

While the "red pill" philosophy has its detractors, it has gained a sizable following among men who believe that traditional masculinity has been diminished in modern society. Whether or not one agrees with all of the "red pill" philosophy's principles, it is an important viewpoint that should be considered and understood in today's world.

The "red pill" philosophy is frequently associated with men's rights activism and the belief that men have been marginalized in various ways by society. This includes issues such as unequal treatment in the criminal justice system, the difficulty of proving paternity in child custody cases, and the expectation that men should bear the majority of the financial burden for their families.

While the "red pill" philosophy encourages men to be open to new ideas and approaches, it also advocates for traditional masculinity. This means that men should be open to hearing and considering alternative viewpoints rather than being closed-minded or dogmatic.

The "red pill" philosophy places a premium on personal development and self-improvement. Not only does this include physical and mental development, but also emotional intelligence and interpersonal skills.

Some proponents of the "red pill" philosophy argue that society has become overly focused on feelings and emotions, resulting in a decline in traditional masculine virtues like strength, courage, and fortitude. They argue that men should be encouraged to embrace and strive to embody these virtues in their daily lives.

Many critics of the "red pill" philosophy claim that it promotes toxic masculinity and encourages men to be aggressive, domineering, and disrespectful to women. It is critical to recognize that, while traditional masculinity can be a positive force, it is also critical to respect others' rights and dignity.

The "red pill" philosophy has also been chastised for being misogynistic and promoting the notion that women are less than men. Proponents of the philosophy, on the other hand, argue that this is a misunderstanding and that they are simply advocating for traditional gender roles and values.

While the "red pill" theory has a sizable internet following, it is crucial to note that it is just one point of view and that there are many alternative approaches to masculinity and relationships. It is important to analyze all sides of an issue and to be open to hearing opposing points of view.

Chapter 2: The Benefits of Embracing Traditional Masculinity in the Modern World

Traditional masculinity has been presented as a negative force in recent years, connected with violence, domination, and poisonous conduct. However, there are several beneficial qualities of conventional masculinity that may benefit both individuals and society as a whole.

One of the most important advantages of adopting conventional masculinity is that it may give you a feeling of purpose and direction in life. Men who accept their natural responsibilities as providers, guardians, and leaders often experience a sense of pleasure and happiness in their lives. This feeling of purpose is especially vital in today's environment, when there are several conflicting demands and diversions.

Another advantage of traditional masculinity is that it may help both mental and physical health. Men who participate in physical exercise, establish objectives, and strive toward them often report improved physical and mental health. This may include enhanced physical fitness, less stress, and more self-esteem.

Traditional masculinity may also foster strong and healthy bonds. Men who are emotionally intelligent, communicate well, and respect their spouses, families, and friends often report having stronger connections with their partners, families, and friends. This might include improved communication, increased trust and respect, and a stronger feeling of belonging.

Embracing conventional masculinity may also help to develop a feeling of belonging and community. Males who embrace their masculinity and collaborate with other men generally experience a sense of camaraderie and connection. This is particularly crucial for guys who may feel lonely or detached in contemporary culture.

Finally, traditional masculinity may be beneficial to society. Men who embrace their masculinity in a healthy and constructive manner may serve as role models and leaders in their communities, contributing to the creation of a better society for everybody. Volunteering, advocating for good change, and having a positive impact on others around them are all examples of this.

It is crucial to stress that these advantages are not confined to males who embrace conventional masculinity, and that people of all genders may embody these characteristics and ideals. Furthermore, it is critical to acknowledge that conventional masculinity is just one component of identity and that there are several other ways to achieve meaning, satisfaction, and pleasure in life.

II. ACHIEVING STATUS

Chapter 3: The Importance of Goal-Setting and Hard Work in Achieving Status

Whether in their personal or professional life, many individuals place a high value on achieving prestige. While numerous things might influence one's position, two fundamental characteristics that are often critical to success are goal-setting and hard effort.

Goal-setting is the process of establishing what you want to accomplish and devising a strategy to accomplish it. You may boost your chances of success and keep motivated and on track by defining precise, measurable, attainable, relevant, and time-bound (SMART) goals. Setting objectives may also assist you in focusing your efforts, prioritizing your time and resources, and tracking your success.

Hard work, on the other hand, is the desire to invest the time and effort required to attain your objectives. Working long hours, taking on more duties, and going above and beyond what is required are examples of this. Hard labor is often required for success since it indicates devotion, tenacity, and a strong work ethic.

Setting goals and working hard may be a great combo for gaining status. You may boost your chances of success and reach new heights of accomplishment by defining clear objectives and working towards them with commitment and endurance. Goal-setting and hard effort are crucial tools for reaching your goals, whether you are pursuing career progress, personal improvement, or any other form of status.

Setting goals and working hard are key components in obtaining status, but they are not the only ones. Education, experience, networking, and chance are all aspects that may contribute to success.

Setting goals and working hard are crucial components of success, but they are not the only ones. Other factors that can contribute to success include education, which can provide the knowledge and skills required to excel in a specific field or career; experience, which can provide valuable knowledge and insights gained through practice and learning from mistakes made in the past; and networking, which can help you build connections and relationships that can open doors and create opportunities. and luck, which may occasionally play a part in success even if it is not directly controllable.

It is critical to remember that success is often the consequence of a mix of circumstances, and that no one aspect guarantees success. You may boost your chances of success and accomplish your objectives by concentrating on goal-setting and hard effort, as well as fostering other crucial skills and attributes such as education, experience, and networking.

Goal-setting is an ongoing activity, not a one-time event. It is critical to evaluate and amend your objectives on a regular basis to ensure that they are still relevant and feasible, and to alter your strategy as required.

Working hard does not always imply working long hours every day. It is critical to strike a balance between work and other elements of life, as well as to efficiently prioritize your time and energy.

It is important to remember that obtaining status is not the only aim in life, and that many other variables contribute to pleasure and satisfaction. It is critical to strike a balance between work and other aspects of one's life and to prioritize one's objectives and ideals appropriately.

It is equally critical to understand that obtaining status is not synonymous with achieving success. Success may be defined in a variety of ways, and it does not always imply earning great levels of prestige or recognition.

While goal-setting and hard effort are vital, so is flexibility and adaptability. There will almost certainly be setbacks and hurdles along the road, and it is critical to be ready to change your strategy and approach as necessary.

It is important to be persistent and not give up on your objectives, but it is also critical to be realistic and realize when it is time to rethink your goals or take an alternative route.

Chapter 4: Strategies for Building a Strong Personal Brand and Reputation

Building a strong personal brand and reputation is critical for both personal and professional success in today's competitive environment. A personal brand is the picture or impression of yourself that others have based on your abilities, beliefs, and personality. A strong personal brand may assist you in standing out from the crowd, gaining reputation and trust, and attracting chances and support.

There are several ways you may use to establish a strong personal brand and reputation, including:

- **Create your own brand by**: The first step in developing a strong personal brand is defining who you are and what you stand for. Identifying your distinctive abilities, beliefs, and personality qualities, as well as establishing a clear message or "elevator pitch" that expresses your brand to others, are all part of this process.

- **Maintain consistency**: Building a great personal brand requires consistency. This includes always presenting oneself professionally, always following through on your commitments, and always living up to your ideals.

- **Communicate effectively**: Building a great personal brand requires excellent communication. This involves utilizing suitable language and tone, as well as tailoring your message to your audience.

- **Develop strong ties**: Developing strong relationships is an essential aspect of developing a great personal brand. This involves networking, connecting with others, and cooperating with them.

- **Manage your online presence**: Your online presence is a vital aspect of your personal brand in today's digital era. This involves taking care of your social life.

- **Exhibit expertise**: It is critical to demonstrate your competence in your subject in order to gain credibility and confidence. This might involve getting appropriate education and training, maintaining current industry advancements, and sharing your expertise with others via speaking, writing, or other types of content production.

- **Take the initiative**: Developing a great personal brand and reputation sometimes means taking the initiative and being proactive. Seeking out new possibilities, taking on greater duties, and being prepared to accept risks are all examples of this.

- **Seek feedback**: It is critical to consistently develop and evolve in order to establish a strong personal brand. Seeking feedback from others may assist you in identifying areas for growth as well as providing useful insights into your strengths and limitations.

- **Be adaptive and flexible**: Developing a strong personal brand and reputation necessitates being open to change and adjusting to new situations. This involves being open to learning from your failures, attempting new things, and accepting new challenges.

Building a great personal brand demands energy and attention, and it is important to take care of yourself in order to preserve your physical and mental health. This may involve healthy self-care behaviors like eating healthily, exercising, and getting adequate sleep.

Being a good effect on others is an important part of developing a great personal brand and reputation. This might involve being kind, caring, and supportive of others, as well as serving as a role model for others.

Chapter 5: Tips for Networking and Building Professional Relationships

Building professional contacts and networking are essential skills for success in any sector. You may open doors to new possibilities, acquire useful insights and guidance, and boost your exposure and reputation by developing a strong network of contacts and relationships.

Here are some networking and professional relationship-building tips:

Take the initiative and be proactive while networking and creating professional partnerships. This might involve looking for new individuals to meet, attending events and conferences, and joining professional groups.

- Be genuine: Being real and sincere is essential for developing solid work connections. This entails being true to yourself and your ideals rather than pretending to be someone you are not.

- Effective communication requires: Building good working connections requires effective communication. This involves utilizing suitable language and tone, as well as tailoring your message to your audience.

- Practice active listening: Active listening is a crucial aspect of developing successful professional connections. This is listening to what people are saying, asking questions, and expressing genuine interest in their views and ideas.

Following up after a networking event or an initial encounter is a critical step in developing professional ties. Sending a thank-you message, engaging on social media, or scheduling a follow-up meeting or phone conversation are all examples.

- Be open to new chances: Developing professional connections often requires being open to new experiences and opportunities. Taking on new tasks, cooperating with others, and pushing beyond your comfort zone are all examples of this.

- Build mutually beneficial relationships: Strong professional relationships are frequently built on mutual benefit and a shared sense of purpose. This entails finding ways to assist others and forming mutually beneficial alliances.

- Be willing to give back: Developing professional relationships frequently entails being willing to give back and assist others. Mentoring others, sharing information and skills, and having a good impact on people around you are all examples of this.

- Network in a variety of settings: Networking opportunities can arise in a variety of settings, so it is critical to be open to networking in a variety of settings. Attending events and conferences, joining professional organizations, and networking online are all examples of this.

- Foster relationships over time: It takes time and effort to build strong professional relationships, and it is critical to foster relationships over time. Staying in touch, meeting on a regular basis, and following up on previous conversations or commitments are all examples of this.

- Be willing to learn: Developing professional relationships frequently entails learning from others and being open to new perspectives and ideas. Seeking out mentors, soliciting feedback, and being willing to learn from others are all examples of this.

  Respect and consideration for others are required for the development of strong professional relationships. This includes being polite and courteous, as well as expressing gratitude for other people's time and efforts.

- Make connections: Making connections is an essential part of networking and developing professional relationships. Connecting with people who share your interests or goals, or who work in similar industries or fields, is one example.

- Provide value: It is critical to provide value to people in order to develop good professional connections. Sharing your knowledge and skills, connecting people to prospective connections or possibilities, and being a helpful resource are all examples of this.

- Online networking: In today's digital world, networking and professional connection development are not restricted to face-to-face contacts. Connecting with others online, whether via social media or professional networking sites, can be a powerful method to expand your network and meet new people.

Being a good effect on others is an important part of developing successful professional connections. This might involve being encouraging, helpful, and assisting others in achieving their objectives.

- Be patient: Developing professional connections may take time, so be patient and persistent in your efforts. Following up with individuals, remaining in contact, and being open to new possibilities as they emerge are all examples of this.

Maintain and deepen your ties with your professional network by staying in contact with them. Sending emails, interacting on social media, or meeting in person on a regular basis are all examples of this..

III. EARNING RESPECT

Chapter 6: Earning Respect

Respect is an important aspect of any relationship, whether it be personal or professional. It involves recognizing and valuing the worth, dignity, and rights of others, and treating them with consideration and appreciation. Earning respect is not something that is given automatically, but rather something that must be earned through one's actions and behavior.

Here are some strategies for earning respect:

- Be respectful and considerate: One of the most important ways to earn respect is to be respectful and considerate of others. This means showing appreciation for their time and efforts, being polite and courteous, and being mindful of their feelings and needs.

- Be reliable and dependable: Earning respect often involves being reliable and dependable, and following through on your commitments and responsibilities. This means being punctual, meeting deadlines, and being consistent in your work and behavior.

- Communicate effectively: Effective communication is crucial to earning respect. This includes being clear and concise, using appropriate language and tone, and adapting your message to your audience.

- Practice active listening: Active listening is an important part of earning respect. This means paying attention to what others are saying, asking questions, and showing genuine interest in their thoughts and ideas.

- Be honest and transparent: Honesty and transparency are important qualities for earning respect. This means being honest about your intentions, actions, and mistakes, and being open and transparent in your communication.

- Be open to feedback and constructive criticism: Earning respect often involves being open to feedback and constructive criticism, and using it as an opportunity to learn and grow. This means being willing to listen to others' perspectives and suggestions, and being open to making changes as needed.

- Seek to understand others: Earning respect involves seeking to understand others and their perspectives. This means being open to hearing and considering their ideas, and being willing to compromise or find common ground.

- Be open to new ideas and experiences: Earning respect often involves being open to new ideas and experiences, and being willing to learn and grow. This means being open to trying new things, stepping outside your comfort zone, and being receptive to new perspectives.

- Treat others with dignity and respect: Earning respect involves treating others with dignity and respect, and valuing their worth and contributions. This means being respectful of their rights, opinions, and boundaries, and treating them with kindness and consideration.

- Be a positive influence: Earning respect often involves being a positive influence on others, and being a role model for others to follow. This means being a good example of respect, honesty, and integrity, and inspiring others to be their best selves.

- Be open to learning: Earning respect often involves being open to learning and improving. This means being willing to seek out new knowledge and skills, and being receptive to feedback and constructive criticism.

- Take responsibility for your actions: Earning respect requires taking responsibility for your actions, and being accountable for your words and deeds. This means being willing to admit your mistakes, and making an effort to correct them.

- Be assertive: Assertiveness is an important quality for earning respect. This means standing up for yourself and your beliefs, and expressing your thoughts and feelings in a clear and confident manner.

- Practice self-respect: In order to earn the respect of others, it is important to practice self-respect. This means valuing yourself, your worth, and your contributions, and treating yourself with the same kindness and consideration that you would show to others.

- Show respect for diversity: Earning respect often involves showing respect for diversity and inclusion. This means valuing and respecting the differences and unique qualities of others, and being open to learning from and collaborating with people from diverse backgrounds and experiences.

By following these strategies, you can earn the respect of others and build strong, positive relationships based on mutual appreciation and regard. It is important to recognize that earning respect is an ongoing process, and that it requires ongoing effort and commitment to maintaining high standards of behavior and character. Additionally, it is important to recognize that respect is a two-way street, and that it requires both giving and receiving respect in order to build strong and positive relationships.

Integrity and honor are two important qualities that can help a person gain respect from others. These qualities involve being honest, ethical, and fair in all of one's actions and interactions. When a person demonstrates integrity and honor, they are seen as trustworthy and reliable, which are essential characteristics for earning the respect of others.

One way in which integrity can help a person gain respect is by demonstrating honesty. When a person is honest, they are more likely to be trusted and respected by others. This is because honesty is a foundational quality that is essential for building strong relationships and building trust. For example, if someone tells the truth when faced with a difficult situation, even if it means admitting to a mistake, they are more likely to be respected by their peers.

Another way in which integrity can help a person gain respect is by demonstrating ethical behavior. Ethical behavior involves following moral principles and doing what is right, even when it is difficult or inconvenient. When a person consistently behaves in an ethical manner, they are more likely to be respected by others for their moral fortitude.

Honor is another important quality that can help a person gain respect. Honor involves holding oneself to high standards and living up to one's own values and principles. When a person demonstrates honor, they are seen as someone who can be trusted to do what is right, even when no one is watching.

Overall, integrity and honor are essential qualities for gaining respect from others. By being honest, ethical, and fair in all of one's actions and interactions, a person can build trust and credibility with those around them, and ultimately earn the respect and admiration of their peers.

It is worth noting that gaining respect through integrity and honor is not a one-time effort. Rather, it is a continuous process that requires consistent effort and commitment. A person must consistently demonstrate these qualities in all of their actions and interactions in order to earn and maintain the respect of others.

In addition, it is important to recognize that respect is not something that can be demanded or demanded; it must be earned. Therefore, a person must actively work to demonstrate integrity and honor in order to gain the respect of others. This may require making difficult decisions or standing up for what is right, even when it is not popular or easy to do so.

Ultimately, the role of integrity and honor in gaining respect is a crucial one. By consistently demonstrating these qualities, a person can earn the trust and admiration of their peers and become a respected member of their community.

Chapter 7: Strategies for Building and Maintaining Trust

Trust is an essential component of any relationship, whether it be personal or professional. It is the foundation upon which strong, positive relationships are built, and it is essential for building credibility and fostering cooperation and collaboration. Building and maintaining trust requires effort and commitment, and it is an ongoing process that requires consistent effort and attention.

Here are some strategies for building and maintaining trust:

- Be honest and transparent: Honesty and transparency are essential for building and maintaining trust. This means being honest about your intentions, actions, and mistakes, and being open and transparent in your communication.

- Be reliable and dependable: Building and maintaining trust requires being reliable and dependable, and following through on your commitments and responsibilities. This means being punctual, meeting deadlines, and being consistent in your work and behavior.

- Communicate effectively: Effective communication is crucial for building and maintaining trust. This includes being clear and concise, using appropriate language and tone, and adapting your message to your audience.

- Practice active listening: Active listening is an important part of building and maintaining trust. This means paying attention to what others are saying, asking questions, and showing genuine interest in their thoughts and ideas.

- Seek to understand others: Building and maintaining trust involves seeking to understand others and their perspectives. This means being open to hearing and considering their ideas, and being willing to compromise or find common ground.

- Be open to feedback and constructive criticism: Building and maintaining trust often involves being open to feedback and

- Respect boundaries: Respecting others' boundaries is an important part of building and maintaining trust. This means being mindful of their feelings and needs, and being respectful of their rights, opinions, and privacy.

- Be consistent: Consistency is an important factor in building and maintaining trust. This means consistently presenting yourself in a professional and respectful manner, and consistently living up to your values and principles.

- Take responsibility for your actions: Building and maintaining trust requires taking responsibility for your actions, and being accountable for your words and deeds. This means being willing to admit your mistakes, and making an effort to correct them.

- Practice self-trust: Building and maintaining trust also involves practicing self-trust. This means trusting yourself and your abilities, and being confident in your decisions and actions.

- Foster open and honest communication: Open and honest communication is an essential component of building and maintaining trust. This means being willing to share your thoughts and feelings, and being receptive to others' perspectives and ideas.

- Show appreciation and gratitude: Showing appreciation and gratitude is an important part of building and maintaining trust. This means expressing gratitude for others' contributions and efforts, and showing appreciation for their time and support.

By following these strategies, you can build and maintain trust in your relationships, and create a foundation of mutual respect and understanding. Remember, building and maintaining trust is an ongoing process that requires consistent effort and attention, and it is essential for fostering strong, positive relationships.

Chapter 8: Tips for Handling Conflicts and Difficult Situations with Grace and Poise

Conflict and difficult situations are an inevitable part of life, and they can arise in any relationship, whether it be personal or professional. While these situations can be challenging, it is important to handle them with grace and poise in order to maintain healthy and positive relationships.

Here are some tips for handling conflicts and difficult situations with grace and poise:

- Remain calm: It is important to remain calm and level-headed in conflicts and difficult situations, as this can help to defuse tension and allow for more productive communication.
- Practice active listening: Active listening is an important skill for handling conflicts and difficult situations. This means paying attention to what others are saying, asking

questions, and showing genuine interest in their thoughts and ideas.

- Communicate effectively: Effective communication is crucial for handling conflicts and difficult situations. This includes being clear and concise, using appropriate language and tone, and adapting your message to your audience.
- Seek to understand others: It is important to seek to understand others and their perspectives when handling conflicts and difficult situations. This means being open to hearing and considering their ideas, and being willing to compromise or find common ground.
- Be open to feedback and constructive criticism: Handling conflicts and difficult situations often involves being open to feedback and constructive criticism, and using it as an opportunity to learn and grow. This means being willing to listen to others' perspectives and suggestions, and being open to making changes as needed.

- Practice empathy: Empathy is an important skill for handling conflicts and difficult situations. This means being able to understand and relate to others' emotions and experiences, and showing compassion and understanding.

- Seek mediation or outside help if needed: If conflicts and difficult situations cannot be resolved through communication and understanding, it may be helpful to seek mediation or outside help. This can include seeking the assistance of a neutral third party, or seeking support from a professional such as a therapist or counselor.

- Practice forgiveness: Forgiveness is an important part of handling conflicts and difficult situations with grace and poise. This means letting go of resentment and anger, and being willing to move forward and rebuild trust.

- Keep an open mind: An open mind is an important tool for handling conflicts and difficult situations. This means being willing to consider different perspectives and viewpoints, and being open to finding solutions that meet the needs and interests of all parties involved.

- Focus on the issue at hand: When handling conflicts and difficult situations, it is important to focus on the issue at hand and avoid getting sidetracked by personal attacks or unrelated matters. This can help to keep the conversation productive and focused on finding a resolution.

- Take breaks if needed: If conflicts and difficult situations become overwhelming or emotionally charged, it can be helpful to take a break and regroup. This can allow for time to calm down and gather one's thoughts, and can help to prevent the situation from escalating further.

- Seek support: It can be helpful to seek support from friends, family, or a professional counselor or therapist when handling conflicts and difficult situations. Having someone to talk to and receive guidance from can be a valuable resource for finding perspective and finding healthy ways to cope with challenging situations

By following these tips, you can handle conflicts and difficult situations with grace and poise, and maintain healthy and positive relationships. Remember, conflicts and difficult situations are a natural part of life, and it is important to approach them with patience and understanding in order to find resolution and move forward.

IV. FINDING HAPPINESS

Chapter 9: The Connection between Traditional Masculinity and Happiness

There is ongoing debate about the relationship between traditional masculinity and happiness. Some argue that traditional masculinity, with its emphasis on strength, stoicism, and independence, can be harmful to men's mental health and well-being, while others believe that it can be a source of strength and satisfaction.

One aspect of traditional masculinity that may impact happiness is the pressure to conform to certain gender roles and expectations. These expectations can include being the breadwinner, being emotionally stoic, and avoiding vulnerability. These pressures can create feelings of inadequacy and stress, and may contribute to feelings of unhappiness.

On the other hand, some proponents of traditional masculinity argue that it can provide men with a sense of purpose and direction, and can be a source of strength and resilience. For example, traditional masculine values such as hard work, responsibility, and self-reliance may provide a sense of accomplishment and satisfaction.

It is important to recognize that traditional masculinity is not a monolithic concept, and that there is diversity within the experiences and beliefs of those who identify with it. Some men may find fulfillment and happiness through embracing traditional masculine values, while others may feel constrained or unhappy as a result.

Ultimately, happiness is a subjective and personal experience, and what brings happiness to one person may not be the same for another. It is important to recognize that happiness is not dependent on any specific set of values or beliefs, and that it is possible to find happiness and fulfillment through a wide range of approaches and experiences.

The connection between traditional masculinity and happiness may vary depending on individual circumstances and beliefs. Some men may find that embracing traditional masculine values brings them a sense of purpose and fulfillment, while others may feel that these values are constraining or incompatible with their personal goals and values.

It is important to recognize that traditional masculinity is not a monolithic concept, and that there is diversity within the experiences and beliefs of those who identify with it. This means that the connection between traditional masculinity and happiness may vary from person to person.

The relationship between traditional masculinity and happiness may be influenced by societal expectations and pressure to conform to certain gender roles. This can create feelings of inadequacy and stress, and may contribute to feelings of unhappiness.

It is important to recognize that happiness is a subjective and personal experience, and what brings happiness to one person may not be the same for another. It is possible to find happiness and fulfillment through a wide range of approaches and experiences, and it is important to find what works best for you.

It is important to prioritize mental health and well-being when it comes to finding happiness. This may involve seeking support from friends, family, or a mental health professional if needed, and taking care of your physical and emotional needs.

By considering these points, you can better understand the connection between traditional masculinity and happiness, and find what works best for you in terms of finding fulfillment and contentment. Remember, happiness is a personal and subjective experience, and it is important to prioritize your own well-being and find what works best for you.

Chapter 10: The Importance of Balance and Self-Care in Achieving Happiness

Happiness is a subjective and personal experience, and what brings happiness to one person may not be the same for another. However, there are certain habits and practices that can contribute to overall well-being and happiness, such as maintaining a healthy balance and taking care of one's physical and emotional needs.

Here are some tips for achieving balance and practicing self-care in pursuit of happiness:

Set boundaries: Setting boundaries is an important aspect of maintaining balance and taking care of oneself. This means setting limits on the time and energy you devote to different activities, and being clear about what you are and are not willing to do.

- Practice self-care: Self-care is an essential aspect of maintaining balance and well-being. This means taking care of your physical and emotional needs, such as getting enough sleep, exercising regularly, and engaging in activities that bring you joy and relaxation.
- Make time for hobbies and passions: Engaging in hobbies and activities that bring you joy and fulfillment can be an important part of maintaining balance and well-being. This may include hobbies, sports, creative pursuits, or other activities that bring you enjoyment and relaxation.
- Prioritize relationships: Building and maintaining positive relationships is an important aspect of happiness. This may involve making time for loved ones, seeking out new connections, and cultivating supportive and fulfilling relationships.

- Seek out opportunities for growth and learning: Personal growth and learning can be an important part of happiness and well-being. This may involve seeking out new experiences, learning new skills, or setting and working towards personal goals.

- Take breaks and allow for downtime: It is important to allow for breaks and downtime in order to maintain balance and prevent burnout. This may involve taking regular vacations, setting aside time for relaxation and leisure, or simply taking a few minutes each day to unwind and recharge.

- Seek out support when needed: It is important to recognize that we all need support at times, and it is okay to seek out help when needed. This may involve reaching out to friends and loved ones for support, or seeking professional help such as therapy or counseling.

- Practice gratitude: Focusing on what you are thankful for can help to improve your overall sense of well-being and happiness. This may involve keeping a gratitude journal, sharing your gratitude with others, or simply taking time each day to reflect on the things you are grateful for.

- Find ways to manage stress: Stress is a natural part of life, and it is important to find healthy ways to manage it in order to maintain balance and well-being. This may involve practicing relaxation techniques such as meditation or yoga, or seeking out activities that bring you relaxation and stress relief.

- Set realistic goals: Setting and working towards personal goals can be an important part of happiness and well-being. However, it is important to set realistic goals that are achievable and sustainable, in order to avoid feeling overwhelmed or discouraged.

By following these tips, you can achieve balance and practice self-care in pursuit of happiness. Remember, happiness is a personal and subjective experience, and it is important to prioritize your own well-being and find what works best for you.

Chapter 11: Strategies for Developing a Sense of Purpose and Fulfillment

A sense of purpose and fulfillment is an important aspect of happiness and well-being, and it can come from a variety of sources. Some people find purpose and fulfillment through their work or career, while others may find it through their relationships, hobbies, or other personal pursuits.

Here are some strategies for developing a sense of purpose and fulfillment:

- Practice mindfulness: Mindfulness is the practice of paying attention to the present moment with an open and non-judgmental attitude. Practicing mindfulness can help to bring a sense of purpose and fulfillment by helping you to focus on the present and appreciate the beauty and simplicity of everyday experiences.

- Find ways to give back: Giving back to others can be a fulfilling and rewarding experience. This may involve volunteering your time or resources to help others, or finding ways to make a positive impact in your community.
- Take care of your physical and emotional needs: Taking care of your physical and emotional needs is an important aspect of well-being and happiness. This may involve getting enough sleep, exercising regularly, and practicing self-care activities such as meditation or yoga.
- Seek out opportunities for growth and learning: Personal growth and learning can be an important part of finding purpose and fulfillment. This may involve seeking out new experiences, learning new skills, or setting and working towards personal goals.

- Seek out support when needed: It is important to recognize that we all need support at times, and it is okay to seek out help when needed. This may involve reaching out to friends and loved ones for support, or seeking professional help such as therapy or counseling.

- Reflect on your values and interests: Identifying your values and interests can be an important first step in finding purpose and fulfillment. This may involve considering what is most important to you, what brings you joy and satisfaction, and what you are passionate about.
- Set goals and work towards them: Setting and working towards personal goals can help to provide a sense of purpose and direction. These goals may be related to your career, personal growth, relationships, or other areas of your life.
- Engage in activities that bring you joy and fulfillment: Engaging in activities that bring you joy and fulfillment can be an important part of developing a sense of purpose and well-being. This may include hobbies, sports, creative pursuits, or other

activities that bring you enjoyment and relaxation.

- Seek out new experiences and challenges: Trying new things and stepping outside of your comfort zone can be an important part of finding purpose and fulfillment. This may involve seeking out new experiences, learning new skills, or taking on new challenges.

- Cultivate positive relationships: Building and maintaining positive relationships is an important aspect of happiness and well-being. This may involve making time for loved ones, seeking out new connections, and cultivating supportive and fulfilling relationships.

By following these strategies, you can develop a sense of purpose and fulfillment that brings you happiness and well-being. Remember, finding purpose and fulfillment is a personal and subjective experience, and it is important to find what works best for you.

IV. CONCLUSION

Chapter 12: The Importance of Continuing to Grow and Learn as a Man

Personal growth and learning are important aspects of well-being and happiness, and they are important for men at all stages of life. Whether you are just starting out in your career, raising a family, or approaching retirement, there are always opportunities for growth and learning.

Here are some reasons why it is important to continue to grow and learn as a man:

- Personal growth leads to increased self-awareness: Personal growth and learning can help to increase self-awareness and understanding of one's strengths, weaknesses, and values. This can be an important part of finding purpose and fulfillment in life.

- Learning new skills can enhance career opportunities: Learning new skills and acquiring new knowledge can enhance career opportunities and increase job satisfaction. This may involve seeking out professional development opportunities, taking on new challenges, or learning new technologies.
- Personal growth can improve relationships: Personal growth and learning can help to improve relationships by increasing understanding and empathy, and by helping to resolve conflicts and communication issues.
- Continued learning can stimulate the brain and improve mental health: Engaging in learning and problem-solving activities can stimulate the brain and improve mental health. This may involve engaging in hobbies or activities that challenge the

mind, or seeking out new experiences and challenges.

- Personal growth and learning can bring a sense of accomplishment and fulfillment: Personal growth and learning can bring a sense of accomplishment and fulfillment by setting and achieving personal goals, and by engaging in activities that bring joy and satisfaction.

- Personal growth and learning can enhance adaptability: The ability to adapt and learn new things is important in a rapidly changing world. By continuing to grow and learn, men can enhance their adaptability and ability to navigate new situations and challenges.

- Personal growth can lead to increased self-confidence: Personal growth and learning can lead to increased self-confidence by helping men to recognize and build upon their strengths and capabilities. This can be an important part of achieving success and fulfillment in various areas of life.

- Personal growth and learning can help to prevent boredom and stagnation: Engaging in learning and personal growth activities can help to prevent boredom and stagnation by providing new challenges and opportunities for growth. This can be especially important as men approach retirement and may be looking for new ways to engage and stay active.
- Personal growth and learning can provide a sense of purpose and direction: Personal growth and learning can provide a sense of purpose and direction by helping men to set and work towards personal goals and aspirations. This can be an important part of finding fulfillment and happiness in life.

By recognizing the importance of continuing to grow and learn, men can enhance their well-being and happiness at all stages of life. Remember, personal growth and learning are ongoing processes, and it is important to find opportunities for growth and learning that work for you.

Chapter 13: The Benefits of Embracing Traditional Masculinity as a Path towards Success, Respect, and Happiness

Throughout this book, we have explored various aspects of traditional masculinity, including its principles, values, and strategies for achieving success, respect, and happiness. While there is ongoing debate about the relationship between traditional masculinity and well-being, there are certain benefits to embracing traditional masculinity as a path towards success, respect, and happiness.

Some of the benefits of embracing traditional masculinity may include:

- A sense of purpose and direction: Traditional masculinity can provide men with a sense of purpose and direction by emphasizing values such as hard work, responsibility, and self-reliance. This can be an important part of finding fulfillment and happiness in life.

- Improved communication and problem-solving skills: Traditional masculinity often emphasizes the importance of effective communication and problem-solving skills. By developing these skills, men can improve their ability to navigate conflicts and challenges, and find solutions that work for everyone involved.

- Enhanced leadership skills: Traditional masculinity often emphasizes the importance of leadership and responsibility. By embracing these values, men can develop strong leadership skills and be effective leaders in their personal and professional lives.
- Increased adaptability and resilience: Traditional masculinity often emphasizes

the importance of adaptability and resilience in the face of challenges and setbacks. By embracing these values, men can develop the ability to bounce back from adversity and navigate new situations with confidence.

- Enhanced mental and physical health: Traditional masculinity often emphasizes the importance of self-care and taking care of one's physical and emotional needs. By embracing these values, men can improve their overall mental and physical health and well-being.

- A sense of belonging and community: Traditional masculinity often emphasizes the importance of belonging and community, and encourages men to build strong, supportive relationships with others. This can provide a sense of belonging and connection that can be an important part of overall happiness and well-being.

- Increased self-confidence: Embracing traditional masculinity can help to increase self-confidence by emphasizing the importance of strength and self-reliance. This can be an important part of achieving success and respect in various areas of life.

- Improved relationships: Traditional masculinity emphasizes the importance of positive relationships, and encourages men to be supportive and protective of their loved ones. This can help to improve relationships and build strong, supportive bonds.

- A sense of accomplishment and fulfillment: Embracing traditional masculinity can provide a sense of accomplishment and fulfillment by setting and achieving personal goals, and by engaging in activities that bring joy and satisfaction.

- Improved mental and physical health: Traditional masculinity emphasizes the importance of self-care and taking care of one's physical and emotional needs. This can help to improve overall mental and physical health and well-being.

- Increased financial stability and security: Traditional masculinity often emphasizes the importance of hard work and self-reliance, which can lead to increased financial stability and security. By embracing these values, men can work towards financial success and build a foundation for a secure future.

- Improved physical fitness and health: Traditional masculinity often emphasizes the importance of physical fitness and health, and encourages men to engage in activities that promote physical well-being. By embracing these values, men can improve their physical fitness, reduce their risk of chronic health conditions, and improve their overall health and well-being.

By embracing traditional masculinity, men can find success, respect, and happiness in a wide range of areas of their lives. It is important to recognize that traditional masculinity is not a monolithic concept, and that there is diversity within the experiences and beliefs of those who identify with it. Ultimately, it is important to find what works.

In this book, we have explored various aspects of traditional masculinity and its role in achieving success, respect, and happiness. We have looked at the principles and values of traditional masculinity, and how they can be applied in various areas of life, including career, relationships, personal growth, and well-being.

We have also explored strategies for achieving success, respect, and happiness through traditional masculinity, including goal-setting, hard work, networking, building a strong personal brand and reputation, handling conflicts and difficult situations with grace and poise, and finding balance and self-care.

By embracing traditional masculinity, men can find success, respect, and happiness in a wide range of areas of their lives. It is important to recognize that traditional masculinity is not a monolithic concept, and that there is diversity within the experiences and beliefs of those who identify with it. Ultimately, it is important to find what works for you and helps you to achieve success, respect, and happiness in your life.

We hope that this book has provided you with valuable insights and strategies for achieving success, respect, and happiness through traditional masculinity. Remember, personal growth and learning are ongoing processes, and it is important to find opportunities for growth and learning that work for you. By embracing traditional masculinity and its values, you can work towards a fulfilling and successful life that brings you happiness and well-being.